Healthy lifestyle:

living beyond 100, and stop unhealthy eating

By

Frank L. Saenz

First edition.

Table of content

Do you need to count calories?

- I shall Be Fit

Chapter 4

Modifying your diet may extend your life by ten years.

Chapter 5

Secrets to an extended and Healthy Life

- Avoid overeating.
- Eat more nuts
- Make use of turmeric.
- Consume a spread of nutritious plant foods.
- still be active
- don't smoke.

- Reduce your alcohol consumption to a minimum.
- Prioritize your happiness.
- Avoid constant stress and worry
- Expand your social network
- Exercise greater caution
- Drink a cup of tea or coffee
- Sleep is important for controlling cell activity and for body healing.

Conclusion

Introduction

When combined, these behaviors can improve your health and set you up for an extended life.

What we eat features a big impact on how long we live to be healthy and live as long as you can.

The connection between food and health is widely established, and following the acceptable diet (and mostly avoiding the wrong items) will significantly lower your risk of developing certain diseases and early death. When it involves maintaining good health, healthy eating may be a vital component of our diets.

We are fortunate to measure on a planet with a wealth of wholesome fruits, veggies, and seafood, also as a

sea full of delectable fish. Modern food has also advanced because the rest of the world has. As a result, foods like noodles, soft drinks, and fried foods have increased in popularity. These foods even have high levels of salt, sugar, and fat. While Non-Communicable Diseases (NCD) like Diabetes, Obesity, and Cancer are now at crisis levels on earth, our taste senses have had little trouble maintaining . Our bodies are paying an important price.

The term "healthy eating" refers to consuming a variety of foods in moderation, including both high-energy and low-nutrient items. A "healthy diet" comprises a variety of foods and does not advocate avoiding nutrient-dense foods altogether, but rather consuming them carefully .

Contrarily,"dieting" entails restricting complete food groups or certain food kinds, which is proven to be bad for teenagers .

Did you recognize that a healthy diet should also involve appropriate eating habits (such as eating only when you are hungry and quitting when you are full) and attitudes toward food (such as not categorizing foods as good, bad, or fattening)? A child's physical and psychological state can also be impacted by healthy eating habits and food attitudes.

Chapter 1

What Is a Healthful Diet?

Healthy eating entails consuming the right ratio and quantity of foods for energy, health, and body construction.

Additionally, it entails reserving fatty, sweet, and fried foods for special occasions alone.

Simple recommendations for a healthy diet include:

Consume two portions of fruit every day. How is that the planet doing in terms of healthy eating, eating three servings of vegetables every day?

Even while there are some wellness champions living healthy lives and eating wholesome meals, sadly, as a society we're not doing alright .

Overweight/obesity rates increased by 8.4% between 2002 and 2012. (increase from 58.5 to 66.9 percent).which indicates that quite 50% of the population of Fiji is overweight. this is often primarily caused by an excess of improper meals and a lack of exercise. Additionally, just 15% of Fijians consume the recommended amount of fruit and vegetables daily, indicating a scarcity of dietary intake of nutritious foods, while rising levels of high vital sign and cholesterol indicate an excess of salt, sugar, and harmful fat in our diets.

How much food should I eat every day?

The average adult only requires roughly 2000 calories per day; the exact amount depends on your weight. If you select health over unhealthy foods, your body will many thanks . Just compare this to a healthy 2000 calories and see the difference. and 2000 unhealthful calories.

What is a healthy way of life?

A healthy lifestyle might include things like exercise, a diet , stress management, sleep, stopping smoking, and maintaining good oral hygiene. ensure to stick with whatever healthy habits you may already have. provides it extra thought if any of these areas need to be improved.

Healthy eating entails consuming a variety of foods that provide you with the vitamins and minerals you need to stay healthy, feel well, and have energy. These nutrients contains water,

vitamins, minerals, protein, carbs, and fat. Everyone should get enough nutrition. Eating correctly may be a great way to support the health and strength of your body when combined with regular physical activity and a healthy weight.

Eating healthfully is crucial for you if you've got a breast cancer history or are currently receiving treatment. Your blood supply, your mood, and your level of energy can all be impacted by what you eat. You cannot avoid developing breast cancer by dieting or drinking. We do understand that being overweight may be a health risk for both first time and recurring breast cancer, although researchers are currently investigating the implications of eating unhealthy on both risks. you'll discover how to eat so that your body is as healthy as it can be in this part. Continue reading to find out more about food types, nutrients, the way to plan a healthy diet, calculate quantities, and luxuriate in food without overeating.

Chapter 2

Designing a Healthy Eating Plan

- You must consume a wide variety of foods that are nutrient-dense if you want to maintain a healthy, diet .
- You must consume a wide variety of foods that are nutrient-dense if you want to maintain a healthy, diet .
- Your best bet is to pick the items from each food group that are the highest in nutrients, meaning foods that are high in vitamins, minerals, fiber, and other nutrients while also being low in processed carbohydrates like sugar and white flour. Choose foods like fruits, vegetables, whole grains, lean meat, and fish. you would possibly want to seek food sources

that are organic. (Organic indicates that no artificial pesticides, hormones, or antibiotics were used during the crop's growth or within the feed that was given to the animals that produced the food.)

- You'll probably discover that fresh foods have less sugar and more nutrients than processed items.

Create healthy eating routines.

1. Eat a spread of veggies, but specialise in those that are dark

green, red, or orange (3 or more servings a day).

2. Consume a good variety of fruits (2 or more servings a day).
3. Consume whole-grain products that are high in fiber (3 to six servings a day). Refined or processed carbs should be reduced or eliminated from your diet; instead, specialise in whole grains.
4. Drink low-fat or fat-free milk and consume low-fat dairy foods.Several low-fat protein options are available, like eggs,

   beans, chicken without skin, seafood, lean meats, unsalted nuts, seeds, and soy products. If you consume meat, choose red meat over red meat at least four times more frequently.

5. Reduce your intake of trans-fats (such as partly hydrogenated oil) and saturated fats the maximum amount as you can.
6. Instead of using solid fats, use vegetable oils (such as olive or canola oil).
7. Reduce your sodium or salt intake every day .
8. Limit or completely avoid "junk food," which incorporates items made with refined white flour,

   solid or trans fats, extra sugar, and plenty of sodium.
9. Limit or completely stop drinking sodas and other beverages with added sugar, which are high in calories and lack many or all nutrients.

10. If you consume alcoholic beverages, do so sparingly. When it doesn't endanger you or anyone else, only drink.

Chapter 3

Do you need to count calories?

Many people think that maintaining a healthy weight requires eating the same number of calories as you burn each day, which losing weight requires eating fewer calories per day than you burn. for several people, but not all, this strategy works. it is important to consider your diet if you're tracking calories. for instance Jane consumes 1,200 calories daily from light bread , cookies, and cake. She's not visiting lose any weight, presumably . Betty consumes 1,200 calories daily from lean protein, fresh fruit, and vegetables. She'll likely reduce and consume a lot more nutrients as a result. Calorie counting is merely one

aspect of the weight loss puzzle.

And calorie counting is simply one method of weight loss. Some studies indicate that consuming foods that maintain insulin levels throughout the day, like lean meat and fish, chicken, vegetables, and fruit, will facilitate your lose weight since the hormone insulin plays a significant role in how your body uses and stores fat.

White bread, candy, and sugar, instead of junk food, can facilitate your maintain a healthy weight.

If you're having trouble arising with a healthy eating plan that works for you, you would possibly want to speak with a qualified dietitian.

The recommendations include consuming a variety of nutrient-rich

foods from all food groups, such as:

a variety of vegetables, including dark green, red, and orange; beans and peas; starchy and other vegetables; fruits, particularly whole fruits; grains, a minimum of half of which are whole grains; dairy products, like milk, yogurt, cheese, and/or fortified soy beverages; and a spread of vegetables from all subgroups.

fruits, particularly whole fruit grains, a minimum of half of which are whole grains. dairy products like milk, yogurt, cheese, and/or fortified soy beverages. seafood, lean meats and poultry, eggs, beans and peas, nuts, seeds, and soy products oils are all high in protein.

I shall Be Fit

- Keep your weight in restraint or strive for wellness.
- Restore fun and play to your life by engaging in physical activity a day .

Engage in a minimum of 30 minutes of moderate to strenuous physical activity, 5 days every week .

- The energy you would like to be physically active is supplied by a healthy diet.
- Develop coping mechanisms, like regular exercise, a diet , and healthy eating, to assist you deal with stress.

Chapter 4

Modifying your diet may extend your life by ten years.

Everyone desires a extended lifespan. We are frequently advised to adopt healthy lifestyle habits like exercising, quitting smoking, and consuming moderate amounts of alcohol so as to achieve this. consistent with studies, diet can lengthen an individual's lifespaned

According to a recent study, eating healthy might add six to seven years to middle-aged people's lives and roughly ten years to the lives of young adults.

Researchers compiled data from a spread of studies on nutrition and

longevity.After creating a perfect diet for longevity, the authors compared it

to the quality western diet, which mostly consists of high amounts of processed meals, red meat, high-fat dairy products, high-sugar foods, pre-packaged foods, and low intakes of fruits and vegetables. They found that a perfect diet consisted of less red and processed meat and more legumes (beans, peas, and lentils), whole grains (oats, barley, and brown rice), and nuts.

The researchers discovered that for ladies and men from the US, China, and Europe, eating a healthy diet starting at age 20 would boost anticipation by more than ten years. Additionally, they found that switching from a western diet to the ideal diet at

the age of 60 would extend life by eight years.Life expectancy for 80-year-olds might be about three and a half years.

The researchers also analyzed what would happen if people switched from a western diet to a diet that was midway between the perfect diet and the average western diet, because it is not always possible for people to entirely change their diet. they found that even with this type of diet, which they mentioned as a "feasibility approach diet," anticipation for 20-year-olds could be increased by just over six years for women

These findings indicate that altering one's diet over the future , no matter age, may significantly increase one's anticipation . But the advantages are

greatest if these adjustments are made early in life.

adjustments are made early in life.

The anti inflammatory characteristics of the many of the foods in this study may also help delay the beginning of different diseases and the aging process.

It are often challenging to fully alter your diet, of course. But simply adopting some of the meals that have been demonstrated to lengthen life expectancy may be advantageous.

Chapter 5

Secrets to an extended and Healthy Life

1. Avoid overeating.

There is currently a lot of interest in the relationship between calorie intake and longevity.

According to studies on animals, a 10–50% reduction in daily caloric consumption may lengthen anticipation .The connection between food and health is widely established, and following the acceptable diet (and mostly avoiding the incorrect items) will significantly lower your risk of developing certain diseases and early death.

Studies of human populations known

for their long lifespans have found connections between low calorie intake, a extended life expectancy, and a lower risk of disease.

Furthermore, calorie restriction may aid in reducing belly fat and excess weight , both of which are linked to shortened lifespans.

Nevertheless, calorie restriction over the future is frequently unsustainable and may have unfavorable side effects like increased hunger, low blood heat , and decreased drive .

It is still unclear if calorie restriction delays aging or increases lifespan.

2. Eat more nuts.

Nuts are a powerhouse of nutrients.

They include plenty of protein, fiber, antioxidants, and other plant substances.

Additionally, they're a fantastic source of a number of vitamins and minerals, including vitamins B6 and E, folate, niacin, copper, magnesium, and potassium.

Numerous studies have demonstrated the protective properties of nuts against heart condition , hypertension, inflammation, diabetes, metabolic syndrome, belly fat, and even some sorts of cancer.

Participants in one study who ate a minimum of three servings of nuts per week had a 39% lower risk of dying before their time.

The connection between food and health is widely established, and following the acceptable diet (and mostly avoiding the wrong items) will significantly lower your risk of developing certain diseases and early death.

Similarly, eating nuts reduced mortality risk by 4-27 percent in two recent studies involving over 350,000 people, with the best reductions occurring in those who ate one serving of nuts daily.

3. Make use of turmeric.

Turmeric may be a fantastic choice for anti aging treatments. this is often because of the presence of curcumin, a strong bioactive molecule, during this spice. Curcumin is believed to

assist maintain brain, heart, and lung function also as guard against cancer and age related illnesses because of its anti inflammatory and antioxidant characteristics.

Mice and insects both have longer lifespans after taking curcumin.

These results haven't always been duplicated, though, and there are currently no human trials available.

Nevertheless, turmeric has been utilized in India for countless years and is typically regarded as secure

4. Consume a spread of nutritious plant foods.

Widespread fertilizer consumption, including that of fruits, vegetables, nuts, seeds, whole grains, and beans,

may lower illness risk and lengthen life.For instance, numerous studies show a lower risk of early death also as a lower risk of cancer, metabolic syndrome, heart condition ,depression, and brain degradation in people that consume a diet high in plants.

The minerals and antioxidants found in plant diets, like polyphenols, carotenoids, folate, and vitamin C , are thought to be liable for these effects.

As a result, numerous studies demonstrate a 12–15% lower risk of early death with vegetarian and vegan diets, which are inherently higher in plant foods.

According to the same studies, there's a 29-52 percent lower risk of dying from cancer, heart condition , renal

disorder , or hormone-related disorders.

The connection between food and health is well established, so choosing the proper diet (and mostly avoiding the wrong items) will significantly lower your risk of developing early-onset diabetes.

Additionally, some studies indicate that consuming more meat may increase the danger of certain diseases and early mortality.

Other studies, however, indicate either no connections or significantly weaker ones, with the adverse effects appearing to be particularly associated with processed meat.

These results could also be at least partially explained by the fact that vegetarians and vegans generally value their health more than meat eaters.

Overall, consuming plenty of plant foods may promote longevity and good health.

5. still be active

It shouldn't come as a surprise that maintaining a healthy lifestyle will help you live longer.

You could gain advantages from as little as 15 minutes of exercise per day, like an extra three years of life. Furthermore, every additional quarter-hour of daily physical activity may reduce your risk of dying too soon by 4%.

A new study discovered that people who exercised had a 22% lower risk of dying young.

People who met the 150-minute threshold were 28% less likely to pass away before their time. Additionally, that percentage was 35% for individuals who exercised in more than this advice.

Finally, compared to low-or moderate-intensity activities, evidence shows that vigorous activity reduces risk by 5% more.

6. don't smoke.

Smoking features a substantial link to sickness and death at a young age.

Smokers may lose up to 10 years of life overall, and that they have a

threefold increased risk of dying young. Remember that you simply can always give up.

According to one study, those that stop smoking by the time they are 35 may live up to 8.5 years longer.

Additionally, abandoning smoking in your 60s may extend your life by up to 3.7 years. In fact, retiring in your 80s should be advantageous.

7. Reduce your alcohol consumption to a minimum.

Heavy drinking is related to liver, heart, and pancreatic disease, also as a higher chance of premature mortality overall.

However, moderate intake is linked to a lower risk of varied diseases, also as

a 17–18% lower risk of dying before your time. Wine is considered being especially healthy due to its high polyphenol antioxidant content.

According to the findings of a 29-year study, men who liked wine were 34% less likely to die young than men who chose beer or spirits.

Additionally, a review found that wine was particularly protective against metabolic syndrome, diabetes, heart condition , and neurological problems.

Women should aim for 1-2 units or less per day and a weekly maximum of seven in order to maintain a moderate intake. Men should limit their consumption to no quite 3 units per day and no more than 14 units per week.

It's crucial to recollect that there isn't any convincing evidence that consuming alcohol in moderation has advantages over not drinking at all. In other words, if you do not often drink, there is no reason to start.

8. Prioritize your happiness.

Your longevity can considerably increase if you're pleased.

In fact, throughout a 5-year study period, people that were happier experienced a 3.7% decrease in premature deaths.

In a study of 180 Catholic nuns, the degrees of satisfaction they self-reported once they first joined the convent were linked to how long they lived.

At age 22, people were 2.5 times more likely to still be alive than those that

were unhappiest.

Finally, a study of 35 studies revealed that those that are happy may live up to 18% longer than those who are less happy.

9. Avoid constant stress and worry.

Stress and anxiety may drastically shorten your life.

For instance, heart condition , stroke, or carcinoma are said to be up to two times more likely to kill women who are stressed or anxious.

Like women, worried or agitated males have a three-times higher risk of dying young than men who are more comfortable . Laughter and optimism could also be two essential elements of the remedy for stress.

According to studies, people that are more pessimistic than optimistic have a 42% higher risk of dying young. However, having an honest view on life and laughing can both lower stress, potentially lengthening your life.

10. Expand your social network

According to studies, having strong social networks can increase your lifespan by up to 50%.

In fact, only three social connections can reduce your risk of dying young by quite 200%.

Studies have also shown a correlation between strong social networks and enhancements in heart, brain, hormone, and immune function, which can lower your chance of developing chronic diseases.

A robust social network may also help you respond to stress less negatively, which could help to further explain how it increases longevity.

Finally, consistent with one study, offering support to others could also be more advantageous than getting it. ensure to give back to your family and friends in addition to absorbing their care.

11. Exercise greater caution

Conscientiousness is that the capacity for self-control, efficiency, organization, and goal-orientation.

Children who were considered tenacious, structured, and disciplined survived 11% longer than their less attentive counterparts, consistent with data from a study that tracked 1,500

boys and girls until adulthood .

Additionally, conscientious individuals may have lower vital sign , fewer psychological state issues, a lower chance of diabetes, heart condition , and joint issues.

Conscientious people are more likely to steer successful professional lives and take good care of their health, and

they are less likely to take risky actions or respond negatively to stress. it's possible to cultivate conscientiousness at any stage of life by doing actions as simple as clearing your desk, following a piece schedule, or arriving on time.

12. Drink a cup of tea or coffee

Both coffee and tea are connected to

a lower incidence of chronic illness.

For instance, green tea's polyphenols and catechins may lower your chance of developing cancer, diabetes, and heart condition .

Coffee is additionally associated with a reduced incidence of type 2 diabetes, heart condition , several malignancies, and brain disorders like Alzheimer's

and Parkinson's.

Additionally, coffee and tea drinkers see a 20–30% reduction in their chance of dying young in comparison to non-drinkers.

Just confine mind that excessive coffee use can also cause anxiety and insomnia, so you'll want to limit your intake to the daily maximum of 400

mg, or around 4 cups of coffee.

It's also important to remember that the benefits of caffeine often wear off after six hours. Therefore, you would possibly wish to move your intake to earlier in the day if you have difficulties getting enough good sleep. Establish a healthy sleep schedule.

13. Sleep is important for controlling cell activity and for body healing.

According to a recent study, regular sleeping habits, like going to bed and waking up at roughly the same time each day, are probably associated with a longer lifespan.

The amount of time spent sleeping also seems to be important, with both insufficient and too much sleep being bad.

For example, sleeping quite 8–9 hours a night may shorten your life by up to 38%, whereas sleeping but 5-7 hours a night is associated with a 12% increased risk of early death.

Additionally, getting insufficient sleep raises your chances of diabetes, heart condition , and obesity while also encouraging inflammation. All of those

are related to a shorter life expectancy.

On the opposite hand, an excessive amount of sleep may shorten your life by increasing the risk of depression, inactivity, and undiscovered medical issues.

Conclusion

Although it'd seem out of your control, there are several healthy practices which may help you live to a ripe old age.

These contains exercising, consuming coffee or tea, getting enough sleep, and avoiding drinking an excessive amount of alcohol.When combined, these behaviors can improve your health and set you up for an extended life.

What we eat features a big impact on how long we live. to be healthy and live as long as you'll .

The connection between food and health is widely established, and following the acceptable diet (and mostly avoiding the wrong items) will significantly lower your risk of developing certain diseases and early death.

www.ingramcontent.com/pod-product-compliance
Lightning Source LLC
La Vergne TN
LVHW020526160826
845677LV00015B/3930

* 9 7 9 8 8 4 6 6 7 4 9 3 6 *